Introduction

It has been a very challenging, surreal time of my career, seemingly in trouble and risking my medical license for having genuinely held un-rebutted ethical and safety concerns, for promoting evidence-based medicine and helping those injured by the vaccine, amongst other 'crimes'.

I have lost much sleep over the stresses of the glut of disciplinary investigations but one of my therapies was in writing poetry, often in the middle of the night after a panic attack I seemed to be at my most creative. I find poetry therapeutic and a unique way to express one's frustrations and concerns. After posting 'A Doctor's Despair' the feedback was incredible and people started to send me their own poems that encapsulated their reflections on the Covid times we have all experienced.

I was particularly inspired by the poem that was read by Tess Lawrie; 'Mistakes were NOT Made', written by Margaret Anna Alice; a profound and deeply moving reflective poem around some of the illegitimacies of the covid era and it's emotional impact. Margaret Anna is joined by some other experienced poets in this anthology, you might spot their work, yet this collection of verses shows that neither literary genius nor knowledge of iambic pentameter are needed to artfully express the pain and frustration in our hearts during this time.

I express my gratitude for all those who have offered their precious work to make this book into a poetic historical record of the last four years. I also thank Belinda for collating the poems together, bringing my inspiration into existence. I also express my sympathy, as the following pages contain words of despair, surprise, disgust and a host of other emotions in response to illness, death, social and scientific breakdown, lies and corruption.

However there is also hope, faith, renewal and a stalwart refusal to give in to the perpetrators of evil. Many of the authors are fellow Christians, some having come to find faith in the Lord God as a direct result of the palpable evil and feelings of hopelessness we have experienced during this time.

As you know many medical professionals have been persecuted for speaking out during this time. This collection of poetic grievances shall be rightly used to raise funds to be used to support legal defence of our names, careers, and livelihoods and for similar projects to counter the narrative that's shown in the following pages.

I sincerely hope you enjoy this anthology of poetry as we join together in our experiences of emotional times, unscientific times, censored times and totalitarian times. Let's all pray for a better 2024 and that common sense, ethics, science and trust and faith in God returns to the world where it is so badly needed.

God bless you all.

Dr Dave Cartland

Acknowledgements

To all the poets: your creative contributions have made this book. *You* have made this book! Together our words have painted a picture of humanity that can be shared to everyone, whatever our medical status or political views. A huge thanks to all of you, and the couple of reflections at the end.

Thank you to Belinda Drew for bringing all your work together into a comprehensive anthology of our time.

I would like to thank my patient wife who stood by me throughout the madness, my children for whose futures we all fight for. I thank the Lord Jesus for his Grace and salvation in and through His shed blood and in His name.

Finally this book is for every single soul adversely affected by these unsafe/ineffective jabs and the government policy related to the last four years.

Yours, with gratitude

David

Poet Hall of Fame

Dr Ahmad Malik
Alex Lawson
Amy
Andrea Allardyce
Andrew Horler
Anon (A Poem)
Anon (The Battle for Fighting)
Anon Colleague
Anon Doctor
The Barred Bard
Belinda Drew
Ben Marble, MD
Dr Billy Ralph
Caroline Sargeant
@CeeKingJustice
Dr Chris Shoemaker
Dr Clare Craig
Damien the Paramedic
David Vance
Doctor Dr McHonk Honk - @TheEyes2022
Erika Loch
The Freds - (Fairbrass/Fairbrass/Ward)
Godfrey Bloom MEP
Hannah French
Jacqui Deevoy
Jane Angel
John Dunnit
John O'Looney
June Slater
Dr Kat Lindley
Dr Lisa Hutchinson
Lindsay Green
M Joseph Burt
@mk_hostile17
Matt Hoy
Matt Le Tissier
Margaret Anna Alice
Margot Orr
Mark Attwood
Montgomery Toms
Nazarin Veronice
N Turner
Peter Huge
Dr Rohaan Seth
SK Poetry
Steven Jackson
Tanya R
The BARRED BARD
Wendy Green
William Bloke

Contents

Poet Hall of Fame 6

A Doctor's Despair by Dr David Cartland 11

Mistakes Were NOT Made: An Anthem for Justice by Margaret Anna Alice 14

The Pfizer Prayer by Doctor Dr McHonk Honk 18

The Heart of Cornwall by an Anon Colleague 19

A Sleepers Prayer by Belinda Drew 21

The Truth Will Set Us Free by Dr Clare Craig 23

The World Went Mad by Matt Le Tissier 25

In the Hallowed Halls by Ahmad Malik 26

Mortal Man by Montgomery Toms 28

Rise Up by Nazarin Veronica 29

Excess Deaths Debate Poem by @CeeKingJustice 30

The seven points of resonance – John Dunnit 32

Choices by Dr Kat Lindley 34

Immune Damage Everywhere by C. A. Shoemaker 35

Virus named Fear by Dr Rohaan Seth 37

Inverted by John O'Looney 39

No Mystery by Matt Hoy 41

Remember by Peter Huge..43
We're All Criminals Lyrics by Fairbrass/Fairbrass/Ward 46
The Death of the Oath by Godfrey Bloom MEP................48
I love you by Ben Marble, M.D..50
Unspoken Fears by @mk_hostile17.......................................51
Buon Compleanno, Capo Mio by Margot Orr.....................53
In the Meantime by Margot Orr...55
Three and a Half by Jacqui Deevoy.......................................57
To Stop the Spread of Covid by John Dunnit......................59
Corona-verse by Dr Billy Ralph...61
Here we go by Wendy Green...62
The Deception by Lindsay Green...66
The Battle for Fighting by Anon..68
Future Fears by Andrea Allardyce...70
My Daughters 'New Normal' by Andrea Allardyce...........72
A Viral Villanelle by William Bloke...74
UnCOnVInced by The BARRED BARD...............................75
Zoom-room Communion by M Joseph Burt.......................77
A Poem by Anon...78
Lost by Andrea Allardyce..81
A Grave Coincidence by Alex Lawson.................................83

Thought police by SK Poetry 84
Bottle Banks by Dr Billy Ralph 85
Are you there God? by Hannah French 87
Future Fears by Andrea Allardyce 89
The Scars of a Mask by Dr David Cartland 91
We See You by Mark Attwood 93
Eulogy for the COVID Kapos by Margaret Anna Alice 95
Rewrite by Erika Loch 99
A Paramedic's Poem by Damien 102
You Cannot Break Us by Margaret Anna Alice 104
Different Sides of the Street by Andrea Allardyce 108
Through the Years by Hannah French 111
When a Hug by Dr Billy Ralph 112
Omicron by John Dunnit 113
Blessed to be alive by Amy 115
Resilience by William Bloke 116
War on our minds by Jane Angel 118
First Do Harm by Dr Lisa Hutchinson 119
A Parallel Universe by Caroline Sargeant 121
The Killing Years by David Vance 123
Cell For Sale by M Joseph Burt 124

Closing the Lid by the BARRED BARD 126
David stood up by June Slater 127
Shropshire Boy by Andrew Horler 128
A Poem by Tanya R 130
What a Mystery by N Turner 132
Boo Hoo by Dr Billy Ralph 135
A Visit from December 2019 by Erika Loch 136
Reflection by Dr Anon Doctor 140
Uneasyjet by Steven Jackson 144
About Dr David Cartland 146

David Cartland: Not been sleeping well of late so took the opportunity to write a little poem at 3am this morning.

A Doctor's Despair by Dr David Cartland

The dark days of these last few years,
A new war, no need to fight,
Totalitarian legacy,
A battle of dark versus light.

A new disease sweeps through the world,
The media swelled the public fears,
That broke a generations psyche,
With a multitude of tears.

Day after day the psyops grew,
Of death, despair, infection,
Apocalyptic imagery,
A solution......gene injection.

Locked in, shut down, alone in homes,
The elderly in isolation,
Images of palms on windows spread,
Accepted by the nation.

The fear of God into our kids,
Governments enforced the rules,
The tears of all our children's eyes
Masked up, sent home from school.

At warp speed, solutions found,
Lockdowns, masks, distance, big pharm,
The speed of science, before we paused,
Injections into arms.

It all seemed rushed, corners cut,
Ethics and safety swept aside,
The solution in a Pfizer vial,
'By accident?', we cried.

The harms became apparent,
When the roll-out gathered pace,
Injured, hurt, perpetually ill,
The despair on my patients' face!

Reflecting now I can't explain
The overreach and violence
Displayed by those charged to keep us safe,
But met by colleagues' silence.

Where is the anger, where is the rage?
The public lost their fight,
Our children's future met with apathy,
Darkness seeming to defeat the light.

But when all hope seems to have been lost,
A small remnant awaken,
In isolation a few stand out,
The fire in their souls are shaken.

Against all odds, Against the flock,
In isolation first, against mounting derision,
An army of brave soldiers build,
To fight totalitarian division

There is a hope, there is a dream,
That we beat this reigning fraud,
Stand up, fight on, small victories count,
A critical mass aboard.

It's time to stand, fight back be free,
Resist the great reset,
A new world order nobody wants,
Look back with no regret.

By Dr David Cartland

Mistakes Were NOT Made: An Anthem for Justice
by Margaret Anna Alice

Dr Tess Lawrie read this poem beautifully in a video in March 2023. Inspired by a conversation with **Dr Mike Yeadon**, it is no simple poem but a fully referenced record of the sorry affair. In its original form almost every second word is hyperlinked to a reference. We highly recommend you view the poem at the author's Substack; Margaret Anna Alice Through the Looking Glass, by using the QR code below.

The Armenian Genocide was not a mistake.
Holodomor was not a mistake.
The Final Solution was not a mistake.
The Great Leap Forward was not a mistake.
The Killing Fields were not a mistake.

Name your genocide—it was not a mistake.
That includes the Great Democide of the 2020s.
To imply otherwise is to give Them the out
they are seeking.

It was not botched.
It was not bungled.
It was not a blunder.

It was not incompetence.
It was not lack of knowledge.
It was not spontaneous mass hysteria.

The planning occurred in plain sight.
The planning is *still* occurring in plain sight.

The philanthropaths bought The $cience™.
The modelers projected the lies.
The testers concocted the crisis.
The NGOs leased the academics.
The $cientists fabricated the findings.
The mouthpieces spewed the talking points.

The organizations declared the emergency.
The governments erected the walls.
The departments rewrote the rules.
The governors quashed the rights.
The politicians passed the laws.
The bankers installed the control grid.

The stooges laundered the money.
The DoD placed the orders.
The corporations fulfilled the contracts.
The regulators approved the solution.
The laws shielded the contractors.
The agencies ignored the signals.

The behemoths consolidated the media.
The psychologists crafted the messaging.
The propagandists chanted the slogans.
The fact-chokers smeared the dissidents.
The censors silenced the questioners.
The jackboots stomped the dissenters.

The tyrants summoned.
The puppeteers jerked.
The puppets danced.
The colluders implemented.
The doctors ordered.
The hospitals administered.

The menticiders scripted.
The bamboozled bleated.
The totalitarianized bullied.
The Covidians tattled.
The parents surrendered.
The good citizens believed … and forgot.

This was calculated.
This was formulated.
This was focus-grouped.
This was articulated.
This was manufactured.
This was falsified.
This was coerced.
This was inflicted.
This was denied.

We were terrorized.
We were isolated.
We were gaslit.

We were dehumanized.
We were wounded.
We were killed.

Don't let Them get away with it.
Don't let Them get away with it.
Don't let Them get away with it.

Margaret Anna Alice

The Pfizer Prayer by Doctor Dr McHonk Honk

Pfizer, Pfizer, in you I trust,
Even if my heart doth bust.
And if my heart doth burst in two,
It would have burst much worse if not for you.

Strokes and clots and MND
Are harmless side effects of thee.
Shingles, tingles, death and blindness,
Are products of your endless kindness.

Rapid cancers, chronic pain.
I will risk MY life for Pfizer's gain.
Inoculate me now, against the evil ISIS,
The Russians and the climate crisis.

My rock. My strength. There's none that's wiser,
Than you, my omnipresent Pfizer.

A-persons.

Doctor Dr McHonk-Honk - @TheEyes2022

The Heart of Cornwall by an Anon Colleague

In the heart of Cornwall, where the sea whispers lore,
Dwelt Dr. David Cartland, with beliefs at his core.
In his cliff-perched cottage, where sea breezes wail,
He pondered the skies, strange clouds in his tale.

His wife, steadfast, a beacon so bright,
Together they faced each challenge, every plight.
Her unwavering support, in every scene,
Together, a team, in times serene and keen.

Nearby, a sheep farmer, shrouded in night's veil,
Whispers of dark alliances, a secretive trail.
Their feud, an enigma, deep and arcane,
A story of shadows, in Cornwall's domain.

Cartland, a sceptic of vaccine's call,
His stance, not maligned, but standing tall.
In public's gaze, his views did stir,
Yet in his conviction, he did not waver.

The local doctors, in their wisdom so sure,
Once deemed Cartland's views obscure.
But as illness crept, striking down one by one,
They realized their need for the outcasted son.

Each doctor fell, like leaves in the fall,
Their once-busy halls, now silent and pall.
In desperation, they sought Cartland's aid,
For the wisdom they once dismissed and betrayed.

With a knowing smile, Cartland welcomed them in,
His moment of triumph, subtly akin.
He'd documented his work, photos sent far and wide,
To the shepherd man, his triumph, he did not hide.

In Cornwall's heart, where mysteries intertwine,
Cartland's hour struck, by fate's fine line.
A testament to his steadfast view,
In a world of contrast, both old and new.

So here's to Dr. Cartland, with his unique insight,
A reminder of the diverse paths we might.
In the dance of beliefs, under the sky's grand dome,
He stood unshaken, in his Cornish home.

The tale now told, of Cartland's fateful role,
In a world of many voices, he played his part whole.
A dance of fate, under Cornwall's sky,
Where beliefs and truths, in tandem, lie.

Anon

A Sleepers Prayer by Belinda Drew

Send us back to sleep, Lord,
Give us back some peace.
Tell them all they're not to talk,
Silence! No more grief.
Tell Mike Yeadon to shut his trap,
And then we'll have relief.

Lull us in our cots, Lord,
Help us close our eyes.
Give us back our BBC;
And we will trust the lies.
Make Dale Wigginton disappear,
And that'll clear the skies.

Do turn back the clock, Lord,
Please return our years,
Send those doctors back to school,
And we can block our ears.
Deceive Aseem, don't let him see,
The reasons for his tears.

Bring back to us our youth, Lord,
Times of innocence,
Take from us the sceptics' doubts,
And trust in governance,
Whip Andrew Bridgen back in line,
Dissent just leads to angst.

But Father if you can't, Lord,
Please save us from this mess,
Help us fight the evil one,
And let us have redress!
Have Calvin lead in songs of praise,
To swell our faithfulness!

Open up our hearts, Lord!
Anoint us all with faith,
Call your flock to spread your Word,
With righteousness and grace!
Come! Lord Jesus, back to earth.
To rule; The Prince of Peace!

Belinda Drew

The Truth Will Set Us Free by Dr Clare Craig

Why tell a truth that's hard to bear,
When silence spares you from the stare?
But hear me now, this truth I say,
The silence costs us more each day.

It's fear itself that grips us tight,
Away from what we know is right.
The fear to be the only one
Against the crowd, who think they've won.

Groupthink, a poison, silent, deep,
It lulls the questioning mind to sleep.
But history shows tyrants thrived,
When voices fade, and courage died.

To speak up at first may seem a feat,
But silence ends in bitter defeat.
Once one voice speaks against the tide,
Allies emerge from where they hide.

And if the fear of being wrong
Disturbs the peace for which you long,
Know that missteps help us grow,
And add to what we collectively know.

Face the masses, un-swayed and brave,
Keep truth out of a silent grave.

The risk to speak may seem too great,
But silence is a heavier weight.

Even power must bend and sway,
And yield when truth comes into play.
For the sake of futures bright and clear,
Please speak the truth that all should hear.

Not all can shout from rooftops high,
But to a friend, don't let truth die.
A whisper shared with those near you
May stir the hearts of more than few.

Begin with doubts, a soft approach,
Let queries be your gentle coach.
The time to speak is slipping fast,
Make this moment count, not merely pass.

The courage found in speaking true
Unlocks the bonds of me and you,
And in that freedom we shall see
The truth indeed will set us free.

You may want to talk about our current plight,
Of pandemic waves or political fight.
But try a testament of a higher love:
The sacred gospel from above.

Dr Clare Craig 02/11/2023

The World Went Mad by Matt Le Tissier

The world went mad in 2020, corrupt politicians
and idiots aplenty,

Scientists and experts with their bought off opinions
and orders carried out by obedient minions.

Fraudulent PCR test gave the illusion of a pandemic,
but the corruption amongst the elites had become
endemic.

We were told we were granny killers for not toeing
the line, time is vindicating and I'm feeling just fine.

Get the vaccine they said so you don't get ill, trust
big pharma they said or you're a shill.

But my gut told me don't do it, don't take the
vaccine, there's something not right here they're not
coming clean.

Informed consent was nowhere to be seen, coercion
and bribery was the governments dream.

As time goes by and the vax deaths and injuries add
up, I'm urging the NHS to finally say stop!

Matt Le Tissier

In the Hallowed Halls by Ahmad Malik

In the hallowed halls where healing's art should reign,
A lament unfolds, a tale of ethics slain.
Silent whispers echo, truths left unsaid,
As doctors trade compassion for an ego-fed thread.

Greed's insidious dance, a poisoned waltz,
Where patient care becomes a trivial fault.
Gold-lined pockets, morals cast aside,
In the wreckage of ethics, compassion denied.

Groupthink's shackles tighten, a binding chain,
Individual voices muted, drowned in disdain.
A collective silence, a conformity's shroud,
Where independent thought is disallowed.

Critical minds suppressed, like embers dim,
As conformity blinds, veils wisdom within.
In the absence of questioning, in silence draped,
Ethics crumble, foundation scraped.

A pledge forgotten, an oath betrayed,
As silence, greed, and groupthink invade.
In the ruins of what once stood strong,
The call for healing has gone terribly wrong.

Yet in the heart of this bleak descent,
A plea for redemption, a call to reinvent.
Let critical minds rise, like phoenix from the ash,
To revive the ethics, restore the healing flash.

Ahmad (Doc) Malik

Mortal Man by Montgomery Toms

Unprovoked acidity, coupled with group mentality.
Attack and disarm him,
He's a fascist, a bully,
A straight white man;
Who we cannot ban.

A dystopian stance, an optimistic glance.
A generation of misery lacking in indefectibility.
Never-ending cognitive dissonance,
A silent majority but a small resistance.

I am tired now, running the line of truth,
Sustained by my firm principles but never to be cynical.

Forgive me of my sin, forgive me of my poor
judgements, I am nothing more than a mortal man
possessed with doing the best he can.
Listen to what I say, empathise and make my day.

We are mentally strong, warriors in this mortal coil,
The time will come when we will all lay six feet under
soil.

Fight for truth, stand for your philosophies,
One day the masses will offer their apologies.

Montgomery Toms

Rise Up by Nazarin Veronica

They locked you in your house,
Said you're not allowed to leave.
Said it's in your best interest,
But they wanted to deceive.

When disproved with science,
They just censored it away.
Told you you're only allowed out
One hour a day.

Then they mandated
An untrialled injection.
Which didn't even
Protect against infection.

People started dropping dead.
Including the athletes.
We kept being censored,
So we too it to the streets.

If you can see that something is wrong
Please rise up, rise up, help me sing this song.
They tried to hide the truth, but we were right all along.
Just rise up, rise up, together we are strong.

Nazarin Veronica

Excess Deaths Debate Poem by @CeeKingJustice

'Twas the night before the debate, when all through the house
Not a Tory was stirring, no orders from Klaus.
The excuses were hung by the benches with care,
In hopes that Mr Bridgen soon would be there.

Keir and Rishi were snug in their beds,
While visions of Courtrooms danced in their heads.
And Judge in his 'kerchief, placed upon his head,
Had just settled their brains, that he won't sentence them 'dead'.

When out on the lawn there arose such a noise,
They sprang from their beds, to see Girls and some Boys.
Away to the window they flew like a flash,
Tore open the shutters and threw up the sash.

The Sun on the breast of the new-fallen day,
They listened to what the kids had to say.
"We want the truth about the Excess Deaths"
And Keir and Rishi, drew in a deep breath.

"We can't tell the truth, or in trouble we'd be"
"Just take the dam jabs and in the morning you'll see"
"They're safe and effective, no harms will you get"
"Pharma are our saviours, we owe them a debt"

Now Bridgen knew different, the jabs they can kill,
And make so many people so poorly and ill,
So he'll speak in the 'morrow,
And raise the alarm,
And the MPs in Parliament shall no longer be calm.

The WEF will send orders for the MPs to obey,
Blackrock and Vanguard will have their say,
But the people will shout and ignore all the rules,
No longer shall the powers that ought not be, treat them like fools.

@CeeKingJustice

The seven points of resonance – John Dunnit

If they are stunned by what you just said
And debate for just a moment is dead;
Then they carry on as if nothing is wrong,
You can sense that you have been misread.

If they feel they cannot distil
what you said with honest goodwill
And prime their gainsaying with : *"So what you are saying is.."*
To imply you are mentally ill.

Although it is not what you meant
You are accused of nefarious intent.
Should you show contrition 'cos they couldn't listen
And endeavoured to disorient?

If you find that the goal posts keep moving
In chaotic assays of disproving.
You answer each case, but they just pull a face
In a belligerent act of reproving.

They may even get angry and yell
At the logic you're using so well
A real diplomat would have trouble with that
Temper's a hard thing to quell.

They may even turn on your name
In an effort to hurt and defame
This is the cost when their argument's lost
Do not gloat 'cos it's truly a shame!

In the end they may simply retreat
Without ever conceding defeat
And so a quiet chat has turned into a spat
Next time you should be more discreet?

If these seven verses have resonance
For discussions you've had in all innocence.
It wasn't your fault they went on the assault.
They are suffering from cognitive dissonance

John Dunnit 15/02/21

Choices by Dr Kat Lindley

They told us to fear the air we breathe
They told us to fear the touch we feel
They told us to fear the life we live

But in the corners of my mind I remembered that time
When fear ruled the world and life was dark
So my heart, this time, chose to shine the light
And all at once I saw their desperate lie

The lie was hiding in the faces around me
The lie was burning through the veil of their deceit
But the truth would remain hidden only for a time
Before the chains of despair would fall apart

There comes a time when one must chose
The path one's story will take for good
I chose light and freedom and love
And I hope that one day, one day you'll come.

Dr Kat Lindley

Immune Damage Everywhere by C. A. Shoemaker

IMMUNE damage everywhere
TOTALLY unseen but it is there.
That was the plan
Always the plan.

To deplete the world of choice
Taking away our voice.
That was the plan
Always the plan.

Promising an end of sepsis
But instead creating
"From a needle – Medical Crisis".

The plan
Always the plan.

The elderly so prone
While shuttered in their Nursing homes.
Attack them first
With poison called
'Run death is Near'

It was the plan
Always the plan.

Then ban the known assists
Vitamin D. IVER. NAC
Never to be advised.
To use what works
Would block the prize.

The plan
Always the plan.

Finally, with world prepared
Mycoplasma and Rickettsia
Will be shared.
The youngest now are most at risk
We weep and gnash now knowing this.

It was the plan
Always the plan.

C. A. Shoemaker

Virus named Fear by Dr Rohaan Seth

There was a virus named fear,
left a mark on the world so dear.
Mindless policies left many in tears,
yet still so many look back and cheer
a response to a reported threat,
the true danger that was never clear.

The government aware the mortality 'from' covid was low,
but chose to spread fear of death, from a "novel" virus?...We don't know.
The reliance on positive tests was inaccurate by far,
with inappropriate use of the pcr.
Healthy people constantly worried they were ill,
while those that should have been seeking help remained still.
Told to isolate from their near and dear,
only to turn off their immune systems through increased fear.

The public were not to know
But media and most doctors just went with the flow.
Unquestioning authority,
ignoring the minority,
blind trust in the majority.

Pushing ventilators, masks and lockdowns,
smiles being replaced with hidden frowns.
Children told to save granny,
The way elderly were left to die alone was uncanny.

Treatments being suppressed,
Dissenting doctors perplexed,
Several spoke out publicly they were so distraught,
Yet the GMC's response was to take them to court.
What was the media's response to all this fear?
They could have given more doctors a voice but
chose to smear.

And then big pharma were given the all clear,
to promote their litigation free jabs without fear.
Safe and effective was the slogan
But dissent continued even reaching 'Joe Rogan.'
Yet the jabs were deemed a success,
despite the constant lament,
from doctors requesting informed consent.
Myocarditis, cancers and neuropathies now a
common adverse event.

What has happened to humanity?
It's become hard to separate fiction from reality.
What has evidently been clear,
This was a pandemic of fear.

Dr Rohaan Seth

Inverted by John O'Looney

Dark skies above and sorrow
Dark times of hurt and pain
We fight for our tomorrow
As evil pours like rain

The world became inverted
The plan it was complete
Policies perverted
And we were classed as meat

Our loved ones maimed and taken
Our young before they grew
And leaders all forsaken
Except for one or two

The parents saw their children die
The leaders poison more
A constant fear, a constant lie
This is a spiritual war

For Satan is inside them
For we must cast him out
He has no place amongst God's men
God's men are here to shout

And as I lose my brothers
And pray to God above
To help me saving others
Save them with truth and love

And twisted truths we straighten
And poisoned skies grow dim
Know God will conquer Satan
For love will always win.

John O'Looney

No Mystery by Matt Hoy

There is no mystery that's written in the stars
No need to sacrifice for being who you are
We're all the same, so don't judge me by my name
It's all a joke, it's all a lie, it's one big silly game.
We make decisions from a face that's on a screen
And Our identity is stored in a machine
We're so judgemental of the things that others do
It's easier, it seems to help, that's what we're trained to do.

We are one
So together we must stand
We are one
Side by side and holding hands
We are one
Facing all adversity
Togetherness it where it's at, so let's give love a try.

So no one warned you, that life would hurt this much
They never told you that different doesn't wash
The hole you feel inside grows deeper everyday
You're not alone, don't be ashamed, stand up for who you are.

We are one
So together we must stand
We are one
Side by side and holding hands
We are one
Facing all adversity
Togetherness is where it's at, so let's give love a try.

Matt Hoy

Remember by Peter Huge

Remember when laws protected the people?
When laws caught the villains, not just the feeble.
The Criminal Courts heard criminal cases,
Not victimless crimes with no lawful basis,

Then came Corona, the magical virus,
That turned the Police into Government Pirates,
Instead of jailing the heads of big Pharma,
Allowing their fate to be settled by big karma,

They arrested the walkers, the truthers- brave talkers,
Becoming nothing more than Government stalkers,
No better than evil media warriors,
Keyboard harassment, creating new horrors,

While leaders introduced a world COVID border,
To usher in their bastard New World Order,
The brave they fought with knowledge and effort,
The people they slept, afraid of the red heifer,

Well the brave they have news, that isn't that good,
The sleepers must wake, where we once stood,
But for them it will be a lot more painful,
For they will see that they gave in so gainful,

And threw away their kids' freedoms,
At a time of new Edom,
Another red reference, not yet that of blood,
But that day is coming, modern day Flood,

That the conspiracist Noah,
Standing alone all the bolder,
Knowing the world's fate was arriving,
At a time that the water was fast arising,

But Noah's water is alas our control,
And the drowning is that of their souls sold,
All we can do is try to help,
Through all the pain we have already felt,

And pray divine intervention follows,
Before the Elite the world swallows,
And bravery reaches the people that sleep,
Before Noah's proverbial waters are too deep,

And we all drown – with some in full knowledge,
That we studied well in our worldly college,
Doing all within our power,
While others slept within that hour,

A time of the greatest need for mankind,
And the people that steadfastly remained blind,
Through fear, ignorance or bliss,
Assuring each night with a kiss,

Their children with no choices,
The little ones with no voices,
That all would be okay,
While we all became prey…

Peter Huge

We're All Criminals Lyrics by Fairbrass/Fairbrass/Ward

We're all criminals, We're all criminals
We're all criminals, We're all criminals
We're all criminals......

There was a time when you could speak your mind down my street,
Now that's all gone cos there's something wrong down my street.
It's all signs and parking fines and cameras in your face
I don't recognise this place, oh it's a bloody disgrace

Can't work, can't play
Can't leave, can't stay
We're all criminals
Can't kiss, can't hug,
Can't dance, can't love
We're all criminals hey
We're all criminals hey
We're all criminals hey

There was a time when there was peace of mind down my street,
Now you can break the law before you're out the door down my street.

It's all a sham they don't give a damn they'll twist the words we talk
Then you'll find yourself in court, if they don't like your sort

Can't work, can't play
Can't leave, can't stay
We're all criminals
Can't kiss, can't hug,
Can't dance, can't love
We're all criminals

Hey, we're all criminals
We're all criminals

Can't work, can't play
Can't leave, can't stay
We're all criminals
Can't kiss, can't hug,
Can't dance, can't love
We're all criminals hey
We're all criminals hey
They're all criminals

Composers: Fairbrass/Fairbrass/Ward
Publishers: FAR Songs Ltd/Sony Music

The Death of the Oath by Godfrey Bloom MEP

When did the Hippocratic Oath expire?
Sacrificed on the corporate funeral pyre
Why did physicians sell their souls?
Abandon their most trusted roles
Five years of training all gone bad
For a twenty guinea fatal jab.

Why did Sky & BBC ban doctors with integrity?
Endorsed by the politicized GMC
Deep State it seems is is deaf
To the concept of excess death.

Where the hell is your MP?
Complicit in this travesty
Endorsing spivs in Pharmacy
In pursuit of global larceny

What is the role of Schwab or Gates,
Penny Mordant & all their mates ?
What place do all these people fill,
With their hands deep inside the public till?

Were they really jabbed or perhaps exempt
The whole damn thing to me seems bent.
Turbo cancers, blood clots too
All for what was really flu.

Oh what a dangerous path we took
When Nurenberg we forsook
Sixty thousand paid the tab
For this benighted evil jab.

So what became of 'first do no harm'
& medicine as vocation ?
When doctors' ethics go astray
For Big Pharma's corporate golfing day.

Godfrey Bloom MEP

I love you by Ben Marble, M.D

I love you
so we won't be afraid
fear no evil
is easier said…
than done
thy will
be art
in heaven
dead now angels
wings are spreading
singing songs
we hope & pray
God's will be done
love is the way

Ben Marble, M.D

Unspoken Fears by @mk_hostile17

The Westminster halls quash debate,
Yet the ongoing silence adds more weight.
The MPs know the truth will come out,
The most awake have no doubt.

The elected leaders know their mistake,
Their constituent voters, they now try to placate.
Excuses spew from their arrogant lips,
They hold the party line as directed by their whips.

Data pours in since 2022,
The UK Government are not sure what to do.
They continue with their poker face,
While everyone knows they are a pure disgrace.

The MPs with their politics degrees,
Cannot understand the complexities.
They need Maths and Stats and Logic too,
The true understanding is only available to a few.

The backbench MPs sit and sob,
All they want to do is keep their job.
They hide behind their Covid masks,
And continue to do what the Government asks.

Their fear betrays a weakness deep,
Their jobs, their status, they want to keep.
They know they must keep up this façade,
The awakened public know they are bad.

Marie Curie, a true pioneer,
Could help them with their irrational fear:
"Nothing in life is to be feared; it is only to be understood. Now is the time to understand more, so that we may fear less."

@mk_hostile17

Written by 15-year-old Margot for her grandparents. Her grandfather was killed with a hospital enforced DNR and Covid "protocols" in 2021 at the Royal Free and her grandmother died when she was 10 months old due to neglect of recognition of sepsis in the ER which landed her in ICU then dead 7 weeks later. Please pray for their souls.

Buon Compleanno, Capo Mio by Margot Orr

Happy Birthday, Captain.
How different everything would be, had you not entered the world
Son, Friend, Casanova, Husband, Father
Grandfather
Our tinkerer. Our best friend
How silly everyone else is, using 'was' instead of 'is'
How strange to think this necklace now is mine instead of his
That every clock in that silent study
tick tick tick ticks on
But the rhythm of your strong heart is going, going, gone
I still can't believe that I can't hug you, hold your hold,
hear the magnets in your glasses snap together
Not at my graduation
Nor on my wedding day
not in person, at least
But I can feel you

in the beat of robin wings
and the walk of a stranger (so painfully familiar)

May your days be filled with light, on that endless,
hallowed plane
May you be finally joined with father, mother, friends
brothers, sisters once again
and her
Waiting
for me
for us

I miss you
Buon Compleanno, capo mio
did you make the shoes?

Margot Orr 13/09/23

In the Meantime by Margot Orr

I see you there
Glittering at me
through time and a pane of glass
(the frame is ornate, but it is you who catches the eye)
So close I can feel you
Your soul glimmering
Facets of you catching the light off my mirror
I see the way you held me
Breathing me in, just as I long to now.
Smile, crooked but heartbreakingly happy
Eyes so blue (and yet they say I look like you)
I can see you, recall blurred moments
(but are they mine or just a memory of a story that I now cannot grasp)
You have no idea – no, you have every idea
Of how I long to know you
To hold you
To know your scent, your laugh, your voice
To hear your ring rap the glass of my window once again
But I can't
all I can do is press at the elastic pane between us
between our worlds
until I am on the boat on the way over

in the meantime
I see you there
see those frozen lovelies
through time and a pane of glass.

Margot Orr 13/09/23

Three and a Half by Jacqui Deevoy

Watching rabbits with Dad through the long swaying grass
Made a mountain of sense at just three and a half

But three and a half years further down the line
My deep faith in sense began to decline

Kneeling, penitent, quaking, small curly head bowed
In a dark, upright coffin, no questions allowed

No sins at that age so I fibbed, story-told
Made no sense at all at just seven years old

(The priest forgave me anyway though.)

My dad way back when was full of great jokes
And laughed a whole lot at the moon landing hoax

He told me most days to question it all
So wise (yet still young), he said not to fall

For the lies and the stories printed in papers
Or to worship celebrities and their dark mindless capers

And to turn a deaf ear to people who try
To be something they're not and who can't help but lie

(Like I did that day to the priest in the box pretending to be God.)

So life went on: much of it never made sense
Especially the last three and a half years' events

They stole my dad's life, those years were his last
I watched him fading each day - dying - through glass

One day again soon, I said, we'd watch rabbits through grass
He remembered, he smiled, right there in the past

Then, gone in a flash, I forgot his Last Rites
His sin not absolved, a forever of nights…

(I'm sure the priest, had he been there, would have forgiven him though.)

Jacqui Deevoy

To Stop the Spread of Covid by John Dunnit

To stop the spread of Covid just turn off the BBC!
It glories Joseph Goebbels' creed in its publicity.
Forego the daily newspapers who profit from your panic!
In time you'll find you freed your mind but the feat may seem titanic.

News editors, like playwrights, have the power to deceive;
Take the ' forty minute warning', Jimmy Saville and Orgreave
And countless other cover-ups and fake news that they spread
To cultivate compliance to an agenda, as Joseph said:
"*A Lie told once remains a lie but repeated becomes the truth*"
So why, when told they are immune, need we vaccinate our youth?

Tune in to these inconsistencies! It's proof that Media's lying.
Last year they said vax-passports came from plotters falsifying.
They lied that covid could be stopped! It can only be endured!
Can you believe these vaccines work when truth is thus obscured?
But there is truth the vaccine's linked to full immunity –
If there's side effect or death, Big Pharma has impunity.

Take note which special words are used to 'nudge' us to their view:
'*Antivax, covid denier, refusenik*, are a few.
So see! Hyperbole is used to fuel a new pogrom.
Without a jab you're a "*loaded gun*"; a "*terrorist*"; a" *bomb*".
In the Laws of Propaganda this behavior can't be faulted.
And as I've said, this has now led to Goebbels being exalted! *

This has happened at least, once before and well we know the cost!
"Impfen Macht Frei" is the new lie that dines upon the lost.
The vaccine leads to a tracking App; a passport just for you.
An up to date sophisticated holocaust tattoo!

So stop the spread of Covid and turn off the BBC!
The Nazis would have got no power without publicity.
Forego those daily newspapers consign them to the past.
Without this fuel they cannot rule and the bullshit will not last.

John Dunnit 04/03/21

Goebbels - "Propaganda must facilitate the displacement of aggression by specifying the targets for hatred"

Corona-verse by Dr Billy Ralph

Spring sunshine brings out the canines with their owners leashed to the ideology of fear.

They happily sniff each others bums as the licence holder looks on in envy and remembers past freedoms.

Two meters they stand apart, the depth of a grave, as they charges tumble over each other yelping with glee.

The dogless elderly long to follow into that vertical void.

The scent of wild flowers is wasted this year as masked automatons trundle by and their dogs pee on nature's efforts.

The evening stretch draws them away from the menacing media and their pooches reveal to them the world as it should be.

Now owners are home all day, no more pining or eating the sofa, a family once again.

Dr Billy Ralph

Here we go by Wendy Green

Father
who art in Heaven.
I pray for all those lying ill
Who don't know the reason why.
Please wake them up to realise
Who has planned for them to die.

It is hard enough for those awake
To comprehend the evil.
The illness spread throughout your world
By vaccine fuelled needles.

So many have had heart attacks,
So many cancer patients.
The end of life protocol.
Administered throughout the nations.

Young men with myocarditis,
That damages their hearts.
The wicked social distancing
That kept families apart.

So many people still asleep.
Heads buried in the sand.
Their eyes and ears tightly closed
To what's happening in their land.

Christianity forgotten,
And evil rules the roost.
People still present an arm,
To have yet another boost.

Immune systems damaged
So they can't fight disease.
While the evil just get richer
And clap their hands with glee.

I've heard just in the last few days,
Of more heart attacks and cancer.
Death rates soaring through the roof,
But no-one tells the answer.

When people find out all the lies,
To make them take the jab,
They will need help mentally
And spend time inside re-hab.

I don't know when the truth will out.
We will be needed that's for sure.
I pray that we who are awake
Will be able to find a cure.

To reverse all the damage
On those still left alive.
For many it will be too late
Too many won't survive.

Some killed by Midazolam
A drug given on death row.
Accompanied by Morphine.
How could they sink so low.

No food or water given.
Just drugs to end their lives.
No relatives to visit them,
Until end of life arrives.

To think hospitals and care homes
Could treat their elders so.
What right to use the Lockdown
Thinking we wouldn't know.

These people have been murdered
With no excuses given.
I just pray Dear Lord because of this,
They are with you now in heaven.

There are many people speaking out,
Against the lies we're told.
For folk to recognise their truth
And for more people to be bold.

We pray it won't be too long now
Revival will begin.
For people to turn back to you
And ask forgiveness for their sin.

To rid the world of evil.
To let the veil drop from their eyes.
So they see your light, not darkness.
Not clouds but clear blue skies.

Amen

Wendy Green

The Deception by Lindsay Green

It was March 2020.
The fear porn was plenty.
The fake news was scary.
The China images made us wary.

We were told there was a virus,
That would come and find us.
No one was safe from this lethal wave.
Our normal way of life now like a slave.

Everything changed to worry & strife.
Our family and friends, fear was rife.
But some of us woke up to the distorted truth.
They tried to break us but we broke through as a sleuth.

No hugs no connection.
The lack of affection.
Just obsession caused by mind control.
The …. programming put us on parole.

We were told we'd be okay if we were sat down eating.
But told we'd face death If we stood up and took breath.

The fear kept on coming it was crippling and
numbing.
Separated from loved ones.
We were stunned and shunned.

We were offered a solution.
An evil resolution.
The Vaccine offered for execution.
We knew it was too quick.
We knew it was sick.
The agenda became clear
It may as well be a spear.

This Evil plan was their plight.
So many good souls decided to fight.
So many prayers said to cause a revival.
It was meant to be for our survival.

A great awakening throughout the land.
God's end game well planned!!

Lindsay Green

The Battle for Fighting by Anon

March 2020, new baby
I'll ignore the news
What if everyone had done the same?

Mania all around, each broadcast giving
false hope – for when had we ever created a jab for
a coronavirus before?
That'll never happen, I thought.

Suddenly! – masks for respiratory viruses. Strange –
my medical school taught the opposite.
People really are taking this too seriously.

We have a jab! We have a jab!
I didn't understand the jubilation. It stank, but of
what?

Propaganda billboards – "Masks protect you! Jabs
protect others!" The message I heard on TV just
months ago reversed. The message's changing! The
message's changing! – But please don't pay
attention. Oh wait, it's changed again!

Families forming, families splitting. Sickness coming, people dying. Strongmen falling, truth exposing, leaders rising. Communities reforming, bodies for healing, prayers for praying, victories for winning, but first –

The battle for fighting.

Anon

Future Fears by Andrea Allardyce

I'm not sure that I'd do it.
If I had my time again.
I might decide to have no child.
And go against the grain.

And not because I do not love.
To be a mum of three.
But what future is there anymore?
What horrors will there be?

They tell us there are floods and fires.
Around almost every corner.
The death species, plants and poor.
Our kids will be the mourner.

And what of jobs and livelihoods?
They say the AI's come.
To help us in our hour of need.
Careers, there may be none.

Watched they'll be, at every move.
Surveillance will make tenser.
And thinking independent thoughts,
Will attract to them the censor.

But what I find the worse of all.
Is how they will be used.

As markets for corporate elites,
Who lie, pollute, abuse.

It's fear they use to condition them.
And deconstructed humanity.
Can't trust their gender, race, beliefs
Or even their own immunity.

For when they are confused and scared,
And suspicious of almost all.
They'll do and take whatever they're told.
And divided they will fall.

For who will have the courage?
To swim against the tide.
And expose these propagandists.
And the truth that they have lied.

Their healthy bodies and furtive minds,
Will be put into the trash.
Genetically modified automatons.
All for a bit more cash.

But what you must guard with your lives,
My lovely children three.
Do not believe their doublespeak.
Your minds will keep you free.

Andrea Allardyce

My Daughters 'New Normal' by Andrea Allardyce

She said in one excited breath…"Mum
We've just had a war.
They destroyed our base, went away,
Then came back for some more."

It's rare we talk, I smile and nod.
And think back to my past.
At last...thank god...I feel relieved.
She's been OUTSIDE at last!

Playing, romping and roaming about.
Being kids, getting scratched.
And crying out.
Perhaps it was dangerous?
Maybe she'd been bad!
But their dens been destroyed.
And rightly they're mad.

Then she continues
To tell her 'big tale'.
"But the server went down mum."

Oh!

I went pale....

"It was a nightmare!
We all had to text.
Took me ages to follow,
Work out what came next.
My mouse hand was aching.
My neck felt so sore.
But we couldn't stop gaming.
We all wanted more."

I frowned and looked down.
To hide my dismay.
"Aren't you fed up online?
Can't you go OUT to play?"

"But I LOVE my new people.
They're called 'Unknown Friend'.
Can't see, touch or meet them.
Just have to PRETEND!"

Andrea Allardyce

A Viral Villanelle by William Bloke

I saw a padlock on the playground gate.
Who on earth will this spitefulness protect?
Remove it now before it is too late!

Where can young love go on its first date?
In Lockdown, there's no place they can connect.
I saw a padlock on the playground gate.

But why can only large firms operate?
Such economic logic is suspect.
Remove it now before it is too late!

I'm worried at the world this will create.
Exuberance is foiled by such neglect.
I saw a padlock on the playground gate.

So, if we let this evil propagate
How can we retain our self-respect?
Remove it now before it is too late!

When will this insanity abate?
Perhaps when all Humanity is wrecked.
I saw a padlock on the playground gate.
Remove it now before it is too late!

William Bloke June 2020

UnCOnVInced by The BARRED BARD

I woke up early yet again at the dawning hour of four
Just conscious, laying half awake, that dread seeps in once more
'Cause COVID rules still plague our lives for reasons stated clear
But their message changes by the day, which ratchets up the fear.

The point I need to clarify is there's 'no stone' they won't assize
As the Government vies to overreach to restrict our sexual ties
I know it sounds ridiculous but partners must now heed:
Don't 'Face to Face', don't close embrace, keep distant as you breed!

As funny as this seems to me, I'm not laughing any more
Cause COVID rules treats us all like fools and there's plenty more in store.
First LOCKDOWN 1, now LOCKDOWN 3, real experts have no say
As social sites scan those 'insights', and ban without delay.

They've killed off education so the kids can't intermingle
Now home alone, no PC loan and a meal means just one Pringle.
Restaurants, pubs and Gyms must close, there's nowhere left for fun
Just STAY AT HOME! And "DO NOT ROAM!" – THERE'S NOWHERE LEFT TO RUN!

And all this time the debts just grow, we're losing homes and jobs
Yet when we protest peacefully fierce Police treat us like mobs.
Now neighbours turn on neighbours breeding homebound curtain twitchers
Where lives are intercepted by keen SS COVID snitchers

And still you can't see Granny though she's had that questioned jab
Those vaccines that they rushed through weren't full tested by the lab.
They call us Anti Vaxx-ers cause we dare to quiz their "Science"

But they, as Anti Faxx-ers, state untruths with great defiance.

W.H.O. changed pandemic guidance helping drive
world based compliance
Yet Boris, Whitty, Van Tam, S.A.G.E all state they follow science.
For 15 years Van Tam had known no evidence that masks work
Then Hancock states "Masks must be worn", with his ingratiating smirk.

As COVID spreads world leaders spout, "It's time to
'BUILD BACK BETTER'"
It's sounds construed, but they all exude this quote quite to the letter.
"Own nothing and be happy" is their edict to beset
That bristles with initiatives they call the "Great Reset".

With fingers stuck in Pharma's Pie rich pickings caught S.A.G.E $$tuffing
The hypocrites, the truthless lies, this time they need handcuffing...
We're unconvinced, we've had enough! Who do you think you are?!
We elected you to be our guide, not an autocratic Czar`

We'll join to RISE AGAINST YOU – WE THE PEOPLE –
WE THE "MOB"
To take you down you circus clowns, you third rate hatchet jobs
We lived in a democracy, our kid's futures now ransacked.
It's time for us to stand our ground, IT'S TIME TO TAKE IT BACK!

THE BARRED BARD Jan '21

Zoom-room Communion by M Joseph Burt

Pizza crust,
The body broke for us,
No wine is mine,
But coffee dust,
Made this cup
From which I sup,
No hands held but the mute is on,
In silence we all sing the song,
The modern Covid lock-down twist
The zoomunion of the Eucharist,
But really I'm ok With this,

Still one,
And our Christ Jesus died for this.
Hold hands across the great abys,
Internet intent,
One in Spirit's what he meant

M Joseph Burt 1st April 2021
For more poetry by this author please see his books:

A Poem by Anon

When Covid drove near
The people were filled with fear
And they held the media dear
Whilst it spoke of fright
And put families in a plight
Not knowing what to do
No matter how they thought it through
No one had a clue.
But many of us saw through
The tales that were told
As the PCR tests were sold
And PPE ran amock
And government ministers made money
This was not funny
As so many businesses failed
With generations of family companies that sailed
Into oblivion .
Many healthcare workers
Were told to become shirkers
Working from home
People were to take a loan
from the furlough system
Not to seek help or yelp
Unless they go blue
And there would be no possibility to Sue
Anyone.
Functional Doctors galore

Could see the roots and more
Of COVID-19
But they were afraid to say
As so many colleagues had been put astray
and Denigrated by the authorities
For daring to say, they knew better
And not following the rules to the letter.
No one seemed to want to know
That there were answers to go
To for improving outcome
as
The government thought that the deal was done
Freedom of speech took a dive
Which meant that many people did not stay alive
Basic knowledge like low vitamin D
Was something that no one wished to see
Was going to help.
This is unsurprising
Due to the issues of vaccines uprising
To the fore
And the insistence of vaccinations for travel
Took some time to unravel
Many brave Doctors wrote letters of exemption
That were made to give redemption
No one could speak out of line
Freedom of speech meant a fine
Hospitals paid for Covid certificates of death
When there had not been a breath
Of covid-19

The first time in mankind
That Pharmaceuticals were used blind
without proper evidence
and fear mongering with every sentence.
Part of the fourth industrial revolution
Or so they say.

Anon

Lost by Andrea Allardyce

I've lost something important.
My future hopes are gone.
I think that I've been broken.
It's all upside down and wrong.

I tried to keep them healthy with,
Food nutritious, fresh and pure.
And when they're ill and ailing.
Used natures medicines to cure.

I taught them to think freely.
Be brave, compassionate and kind.
Tread lightly upon their planet.
And always respect their mind.

And now they're grown and full of life.
They're vital and they're bright.
Our futures are in all their hands
We need them to exude light.

Instead they will be muzzled.
Conditioned to believe,
That they pose a deadly threat to all,
Every time they breathe.

Their vital oxygen sats reduced
They will not see expression.
But visible to them daily.
Are these symbols of oppression.

Of course there is no evidence.
That masks prevent infection.
But to avoid the harms they cause.
They'll accept an experimental injection.

Brand new mRNA technology,
Will course through every part,
Of their young and health bodies.
Causing damage to their heart.

But worse than any physical harm,
Will be weakness and reliance.
On instructions from the corporatocracy,
Imprisoned by their compliance.

For them is why we stand and fight.
With God, slings and our free mind.
Against the fascist, enslavers.
For the future of human kind.

Andrea Allardyce

A Grave Coincidence by Alex Lawson

As people queue up at the behest of the 'man',
Voluntarily injecting poisons that can
Affect how we live, both now and tomorrow,
Creating a future of enslavement and sorrow.
Considered 'experimental' by the shills at the WHO,
Inducing reactions that forever change you.
NO! to your passports, restrictions and tests,
Every one of us here can decide what is best.
Guinea pigs sacrificed, virtue led fools,
Entranced by their leaders and propaganda tools.
Nobody knows how the ADR's will accrue,
Of side effects worse than this 'seasonal flu'.
Can you imagine life when the roll out is done,
Including the children if their parents succumb.
Denial, obfuscation, nothing left to say,
Except if we rise as one, and do not obey.

Research…

Alex Lawson 30/10/2023

Thought police by SK Poetry

The sword of Damocles appears,
Its shadow broad forbidding light,
The hand that hold draped in spite,
Its power derived from system might,

In hatred drawn and compound fear,
With hollow virtue piercing fright,
The loving lie constricting tight,
The steaming pile painted white.

All this against truth to hear,
It cannot stand in open sight,
For hatred hypocrisy cloaks like night,
Imposed unwanted it claims the right.

And now its victim frustration tear,
And rage to grapple kick and fight,
But punching air and ghostly rite,
Their cowardly stature at its height.

S K Poetry

Bottle Banks by Dr Billy Ralph

Bottle banks full whilst churches are empty.

Amazon blooming whilst florists go bust.

Face masks and rubber gloves instead of summer
dresses and flip-flops.

Bums glued to seats as eyes glide across screens
whilst hurleys stand still.

Netflix devoured in silence whilst guitars long to be
strummed.

The old grow lonelier whilst the young forgo their
youth and grow lonelier too.

Walking trails grow fewer and fainter as worry lines
form deeper and darker.

Truth fades as propaganda paints a new reality.

Politicians speak words as substantial as candyfloss
as the electorate gorges themselves and are made
fearful.

Hope is rationed, questions ignored whilst the truth
is strangled at birth.

Cancers disappear to make way for an ancient foe of
dubious virulence.

Science regressed as Galileo's telescope is shunned, again.

Bernays smiles and catches his sneeze to protect the house of cards.

The world is closed but McDonald's is open.

Dr Billy Ralph

Are you there God? by Hannah French

Are you there God?
It's dark and I'm scared

I thought I had studied
Thought I was prepared
I knew about trials
That temptations would come

I thought I might face them
One by one
But they're fierce and constant and raging relentless
I'm not supposed to despair or depend on my
senses

I'm left hoping some roots hold my battered frame
Please tell me Your book still bears my name?
Then I can bear this storm so rough
It would tear from me all that I've heard of Your love

It would shake and disturb so no peace can reside
It would rip up foundations
Do I really abide?
It's dark and I'm scared that Your presence has gone

All I have are the pages Your Spirit breathed on
Who told me to trust even when I can't see
- You will never leave nor forsake me

So please come and find me

I've lost my way
I never wanted to wander
I don't want to stray
Help me Lord in my unbelief

May the light of your truth make the darkness flee
I'm reading the words but fear and shame battle
with the faith I claim
I seek Your will but the strength I can't find

The power to live was never mine
Wasted pain time after time
May my heart now exposed be renewed and
refined?
As the sun rises so your mercy persists

As the world is held so in You I exist.
You are there God
Help me understand

- I am safe and engraved in the palm of your Hand.

Hannah French

Future Fears by Andrea Allardyce

I'm not sure that I'd do it.
If I had my time again.
I might decide to have no child.
And go against the grain.

And not because I do not love.
To be a mum of three.
But what future is there anymore?
What horrors will there be?

They tell us there are floods and fires.
Around almost every corner.
The death species, plants and poor.
Our kids will be the mourner.

And what of jobs and livelihoods?
They say the AI's come.
To help us in our hour of need.
Careers, there may be none.

Watched they'll be, at every move.
Surveillance will make tenser.
And thinking independent thoughts,
Will attract to them the censor.

But what I find the worse of all.
Is how they will be used.

As markets for corporate elites,
Who lie, pollute, abuse.

It's fear they use to condition them.
And deconstructed humanity.
Can't trust their gender, race, beliefs
Or even their own immunity.

For when they are confused and scared,
And suspicious of almost all.
They'll do and take whatever they're told.
And divided they will fall.

For who will have the courage?
To swim against the tide.
And expose these propagandists.
And the truth that they have lied.

Their healthy bodies and furtive minds,
Will be put into the trash.
Genetically modified automatons.
All for a bit more cash.

But what you must guard with your lives,
My lovely children three.
Do not believe their doublespeak.
Your minds will keep you free.

Andrea Allardyce

The Scars of a Mask by Dr David Cartland

The power of a smile,
The anguish of a frown,
To tell someone you're feeling great,
To signal when you're down.

We smile when we are joyful,
We frown when things get tough,
Our faces show the world our thoughts,
Our grimace when we feel rough.

The barrier to this — the facial mask,
The debate of whether it works,
To stop the spread of covid? No.
But yes to displays of joy and fear and mirth.

To see our children suffering,
In an emotionless world of fears,
To see our children reaching out,
A masked child's scars bring tears.

We rely on the power of our faces,
To tell the world we're fine,
We rely on the power of expression,
To show all the feelings of mine.

It's time to lose the facial masks,
For the good of humankind,
So we connect again as humans do,
And display our souls and mind.

Let us see in years to come,
When we hope we've won this race,
The needs and dreams of all the world,
Freely etched upon our face.

Dr David Cartland

We See You by Mark Attwood

The scales have fallen from our eyes;
The veil has drifted down from the sky;
Meandering firmly; finally revealing...
Your depth of depravity, that's fear you're now feeling.

We see you.

Your demonic blood lust laid bare to see;
The statue of filth on the BBC.
The Prince and the Madam, the CRISPR spy;
The Islands of Horrors in the ocean lie.

We see you.

A billion souls, stolen, over the years;
You hid them deep down to drown their tears;
Perfect and innocent, God's own creations;
Mutilated by your sick machinations.

We see you.

Vlad the Impaler and his vile descendants;
Fleeing the Palace from the 5D ascendents.
The virus distracted, but gave us the time;
To peel back the layers of your heinous crimes.

We see you.

Run, run, as fast as you can;
Back for more orders from the Phoenician clan;
Out of white rabbit, the looking glass cracked;
Tipping point reached, odds against you now
stacked.

We see you.

Pizza and hot dogs, pasta and sauce;
Your sickness decoded your lack of remorse.
Our slumber is over, our eyes not wide shut;
For the children of Haiti, a knife to your gut.

We see you.

Ascension is powered by the light of the flare;
Scramble like rats to the ruins of your lairs.
It's over, it's over, "Save our Children", we cry;
Revealed, reviled, it's your souls' time to die.

We see you.

Mark Attwood

Eulogy for the COVID Kapos by Margaret Anna Alice

"The surest way to work up a crusade in favor of some good cause is to promise people that they will have a chance of maltreating someone. Men must be bribed to build up and do good by the offer of an opportunity to hurt and pull down. To be able to destroy with a good conscience, to be able to behave badly and call your bad behavior 'righteous indignation'—this is the height of psychological luxury, the most delicious of moral treats."
—Aldous Huxley, Introduction (July 24, 1933) to Samuel Butler's *Erewhon*, Easton Press (1934)

You mocked us.
You blocked us.
You wished for our deaths.

You shamed us.
You blamed us.
You called for our jailing.

You banned us.
You canned us.
You cut off our funds.

You believed.
You decreed.
You complied.

You denied.

You feared.
You sneered.
You cowered.
You lied.

You followed the leader.
You chanted the slogans.

You balked at our questions.
You scoffed at our research.

You thought you were smarter.
You felt you were safer.
You knew you were holier.
You said you were better.

Now you're starting to wonder.
Now you're starting to doubt.
Now you're starting to remember.
Now you're regretting.

You can't undo what you've done to yourself.
You can't undo what you've done to your loved ones.
You can't undo what you've done to us.
You can't undo what you've done to the world.

And now you want a mulligan.
Now you want to forget.
Now you want *us* to forget.

Even though it's still happening.
Even though we're still suffering.
Even though they're still murdering.

It will never end without acknowledgment.
It will never end without accountability.
It will never end without remorse.
It will never end without justice.

So make your apologies,
  and we may listen.
Make your amends,
  and we may forgive.
Make your peace,
  and we may accept.

Or not.

It all depends
  on you.

Your sincerity.
Your willingness to take responsibility.
Your ability to name your wrongs.
Your actions to rectify what's been done—

what they've done,
what you've done,
what they're trying to do.

How do you know you won't fall for the next one?
How do you know you won't line up for more?
How do you know you won't crumble again?

Who were you then?
Who are you now?
Who will you become?
Why should we trust you?

Can you see it?
Can you say it?
Can you feel it?
Will you stop it?

Margaret Anna Alice

Rewrite by Erika Loch

Like a crane hit to the brain, and a car crash through the heart
When we face the Truth, distilled – all aligns to North.
If you let it move you, even when you cannot move
When we allow its sovereign call, there will come new shores.

And many will try and tell them, that we knew it all along
But what good will that do when what they didn't know has gone?
Could we be the Ones to say it's time to change the song?

For We will bring new anthems, and commute the ones who stole the stars
It may feel cold and baron, for a while – the tracks of justice healed through our scars.
To bear it as our souls grow, and when we surrender, let go
Of the truth we thought was real before when it's not about that, anymore.

Because all will be known, and all will be true
From the bottoms and up through our hearts
That are no longer tainted, no longer starved
Of the light we had all along
Had we not been played like a song,
Into hand. And stopped thinking.

And still, We were always the stars.

Even when we drank too much and when we lost our way
Even when we went too far, we swerved the devil, and his play.
So join, and rise, and love in faithdom, for His strength we pray
Then build, and cherish, bring forth the skies because this pain is not to stay.

New art will be born
We'll remember. And grieve.
And We will create new life
One free of thrones, districts and zones – and an age not stolen by thieves.
And it will be Beauty, if we can co-fathom
A playbook without blood and stones.

Breathe it and feel it and know it and be it
Throughout the storms of each day
Come the darkness, we can see it
Come the darkness, we will meet it
As it melts itself away.

The cries from the cuts from the ties to the lies,
All the stories that led us astray
And even the darling ones, so long loved,
those, too, they cannot stay.

The poems that we paint
And the melodies that we make
All the artists writing in the now
And to the digital soldiers, like none before you,
The Seekers not in it for the bow.

The new stars will be different, not born of a system
Begun with blood on its hands
Set up to conquer
Set up to make darker
Set up to slaughter the lambs.

And still, We were always the stars.

To The Ultimate Band
The Band of All Time
With a chorus I can't yet explain
We'll write it one day, in harmony we'll play
And this time it won't be in vain.
Wiser of mind and Younger of heart
Each step begins a start
We write it each day, its well underway
With a strum on a global guitar
To The Ultimate Band
To The Band of All Time
Sing a lullaby to sky and terrain
United this day, swords put down to lay
In the rightest most glorious rain.

Erika Loch

A Paramedic's Poem by Damien

I need to ask, have things always been corrupt?
Concocted response times that the bosses instruct
Yes they routinely fiddle the figures'
Through tactics a plenty they lie with such vigour

How could that happen, how could that be?
When the Westminster watches and must oversee
No secret to MP's that the NHS lies
In doing so the politicians failures they hide

Why am I talking about response time fraud
In a book about covid, I can hear the roars
Because I've been witness to the rot first hand
I was little surprised when I saw what was planned

So knowing they lie with such passion and ease
I soon understood the agenda agreed
They never cared or considered the harm
Their only ambition was one in each arm

They made children wear masks throughout the whole
day
To be seen to be acting in a responsible way
They deliberately 'scared the pants' off the old
Knowing that soon on a needle they would be sold

It mattered little to whom the arms belonged
Arms young, arms old, arms weak and arms strong

You could've had the disease and be already immune
But somehow they convinced you, you needed it soon

When it came to mortality, illness and masks
All their lies were to achieve this one task
They said you were ill even though you felt well
To get you injected, it was such a hard sell

They made people have one, two and more
With each passing season big pharma did score
They told how a drug that worked so well
Now needed boosters, oh what a cartel

So how did we get to this point in time
Where most know what happened and know of the crime
It is happening and still nothing is won
We must bring those to justice and make it undone

The orchestraters themselves will never admit
Just like response times they will be seen to permit
They'll say it's conspiracy and antivax lies
When they're the ones with something to hide

We go from here knowing we're right
Knowing we must continue the fight
We will not bend, buckle or fail
Because it's on us that the truths prevail

Damien, a Paramedic

You Cannot Break Us by Margaret Anna Alice

"Nothing gives one person so great advantage over another, as to remain always cool and unruffled under all circumstances."
—Thomas Jefferson, Letter to Francis Eppes, May 21, 1816

You can target us.
You can bully us.
You can fear-bomb us.
You can scold us.

You can name-call us.
You can gaslight us.
You can banish us.
You can troll us.

You can promulgate lies.
You can even believe those lies.

But it doesn't make them true.
No matter what you think.
No matter what you feel.
No matter what you do.

Our words speak for themselves.
Our character speaks for itself.
Our love speaks for itself.

You can shun us.
You can shame us.
You can shove us.
You can shackle us.

You can slight us.
You can spite us.
You can strip us.
You can stomp us.

Your whispering only makes you louder.
Your sneaking only makes you rasher.
Your bludgeoning only makes you bloodier.

You can malign us.
You can muffle us.
You can mandate us.
You can mothball us.

You can declaw us.
You can defrock us.
You can debank us.
You can delete us.

Your arrows only fill our quiver.
Your barbs only sharpen our thinking.
Your slashes only craft our kintsugi.

You can sully us.
You can splinter us.
You can segregate us.
You can sever us.

You can abuse us.
You can accuse us.
You can assault us.
You can administer us.

Your hatred only makes us love more.
Your darkness only makes us light more.
Your malevolence only makes us brave more.

You can disarm us.
You can detain us.

You can demonize us.
You can decimate us.

You can indoctrinate our children.
You can injure our children.
You can iatrogenocide our children.
You can inter our children.

But you cannot break us.
You cannot break us.
You cannot break us.

You *will* not break us.

Margaret Anna Alice

Different Sides of the Street by Andrea Allardyce

We live in the same neighbourhood,
Our lives almost identical.
Across the road a parallel universe,
Where all is now nonsensical.

Educated and affluent,
With a decent and open mind.
Both engaged in the narrative,
How can you be so blind?

We look at the same images,
Clever illusions that hide a sin.
You just see the pretty pictures,
Not the messages hidden within.

I can't unsee this horror,
Now the curtain has been lifted.
All that made sense to me before
Normality forever shifted.

Our government doesn't serve us,
Transparency they detest.
They lie, obfuscate and deceive,
Puppets of corporate interest.

'The scientists'; all-knowing and correct,
No matter what the contrary data.
Must not be questioned or maligned,
By a flat-earther, extreme-right, hater.

Medical experiments, the stuff of nightmares,
Even children are not spared.
Efficacy, necessity, unimportant.
Safety red-flags never shared.

Regulatory bodies meant to protect,
Have all been bribed and bought.
No matter how much damage is done
They know they won't get caught.

Trusted supranational organisations,
We learn are the puppet masters.
Populated by wealthy elites, psychopaths,
Megalomaniacs and bastards.

They're buying all the fertile land,
And stopping the farmers grow.
So were forced to buy; toxic, synthetic food.
Most people will never know.

They're taking away our freedom.
Our ability to move around,
Our once peaceful and sovereign country.
15-minute cities imprisoned and bound.

Tracked and traced, chipped and pined,
The all-seeing eyes upon us.
Genetically modified and digitally logged.
Who will dare make a fuss.

For anyone who is brave enough,
To shout that this is wrong.
Is cancelled, abused or disappeared,
By the righteous, brainwashed throng.

Words and history manipulate and censored,
So that we can't express.
What use to be obvious to us all,
We're a divided, confused mess.

Whilst the control grid tightens daily,
Our media's missing in action.
Information carefully selected,
To give the perfect distraction.

I wish that I could cross back,
To the other side of the street.
Shut my ears and close my eyes,
So old friends again could meet.

Andrea Allardyce

Through the Years by Hannah French

Most of the years
Given to me
Spent unable to see
Each day of waste
Cannot be replaced
Or taken back
The rest of my years
Given into your hands
Now I understand
Today is a chance
To live my life for you
I give it back
These years You prepare
Mansions fair
For hearts lost to the world
No tomorrow disturbs
Waiting for You
To come back.

Hannah French

When a Hug by Dr Billy Ralph

When a hug or a handshake become alien gestures used only by the senile or intellectually impaired, who then is really awake?

When gathering on the banks of the canal to bathe in the sunlight and glory of one's fleeting youth is an 'appalling' vista, for whom are we building a society?

When medical autocracy and political complicity negate bodily integrity, why have a republican constitution?

When once respected purveyors of news become mere advertisers of products and government catchphrases, why have an education system?

When those who have sworn to uphold the law mindlessly beat and fine their fellow citizens, why have a police force?

When the medical profession earn vast sums of money for not seeing patients or obtaining informed consent, why trust them anymore?

When scientists lie in the service of self and state at the expense of our freedoms and souls, why do we listen to them?

When decency, love, contact and gathering become weapons of death, why live anymore?

Dr Billy Ralph

Omicron by John Dunnit

Omicron? Or is it zero micron?
You terrifying tiny germ!
You monster immeasurable infinitesimal.
You abysmal dragon worm?

Unseen, you are feared the most
By shadow frightened fools, who boast
They mask up for the benefit of all
And stand apart in defiance of a threat so small
As to not exist at all.

And so, they cast their civic dues
Into your crucible of fiction. Queues
Of these selfish martyrs skewed by Cyprian Science,
Sacrifice their precious children in forlorn compliance
To gross corruption
Made manifest by vile behaviourists' mass induction.

Omicron you're not unique!
You are second hand and weak!
Just a script: oblique and underhand
Vomiting across this land;
Preached by dupes, toadies, traitors and knaves
False media idols and political puppets. Slaves

That destroy our world with the letters of their law.
"Build back Better" – they cry – better than how it was before?

Really? Better for who? For me? Unlikely!
And to build back better first you must destroy
That which is unsightly.
Omicron you're just a ploy:

A contrivance; a gambit of globalists' greed.
To shut down the world economy and seed
Their diabolical Deuteronomy -
Those laws of conduct for their promised land.

And what land is promised? Rather, what is planned
For the rest of us? "You will own nothing and be
happy."
So, says that world economic forum chappy Klaus.
Or Santa Klaus the Globalists' hero
Author of 'The Great Reset' who, like a Nero
Wants to burn the Earth for Baphomet
and attend the New World Order's birth.

Omicron you are just a champion of sleaze!
These Plutocrats are the real disease.
They call us sheep and "useless eaters"
To be thinned out; culled by their servile cheaters
And you Omicron? You are a sham.
Derisorily named as an anagram
Profoundly callous and crassly ironic
So, all who accept you, like you, are MORONIC!

John Dunnit 16/12/21

Blessed to be alive by Amy

We knew they were no good for you
We just wanted to help
We cried and cried and cried some more
We are not made of skelp

We hoped you'd listen to our cries
We wished and prayed for you
We sincerely only ever cared
We hoped you'd see that too

We still are fighting every day
We will not ever stop
We are all so blessed to be alive
We see through the psy-op

We plea and beg you one more time
To look a little more
Our hearts will all beat as one
As we march on for this cause

Amy, June 2022

Resilience by William Bloke

Behold! I am still here.
Despite the anger, grief and despite the pain.
I am still here!
I march in soft hope over dissonant rills,
Hated, but I endure disdain.

I have sailed many tempests but am still here.
Flushed upon forsaken shores,
I grabbed life from fleeting chance,
As ever to find new purpose.
Then truly, I say: "I've been here before".

So, if you need me, I will still be here,
And if you say not, then I will wait
For you to rouse from slumbers.
Yet resolutely, I am still here
For me, for you, I remonstrate!

For you my comrades, I am still here.
Our differences fill our sails
And glide us to some sun brinded Isle
That shimmers, just out of view.
As One, we tack past what prevails.

As One, and as many ones
As trudge alone in shy tenacity,
Asserting: "*We are still here and free*"!
Synchronised in stoic chorus.
Together, an amassment of audacity.

We the Guardians, of unyielding Truth.
A single taper in the brooding dark
The ignition of truth's brilliance
to incinerate the diabolic plan.
We are still here.
We are His anthem to resilience.

William Bloke January 2023

Wonderful words like: 'resilience' have been repurposed for nefarious schemes by psychopathic ghouls. I want to rescue them from their dark confinements and bring them back into the light.

War on our minds by Jane Angel

All under a spell not having a clue
Sole focus on the virus, what it can do to you!
Immoral mind methods used to control,
the fear, the trauma, taking its toll.

They terrified the masses, not caring one bit.
Many innocent groups taking the hit.
Nudges, no ethics were clearly discussed,
To get your obedience was an absolute must.

Persuasion, coercion, it didn't matter at all.
They wanted you cowering not standing tall
Our elders too frightened to step out the door
A continual attack on the mind, a war.

Folk hysterical at the sight of a face,
All by design this was the case
Where was consent, we didn't give it.
Nobody did, we were just forced to live it…

Jane Angel

First Do Harm by Dr Lisa Hutchinson

Behind the establishment veil of lies
Lurks the new world order in disguise
Normal existence, a disturbing mantra of fear
Democratic values, a distant memory my dear

Hippocratic Oath states "First Do No Harm"
Reality of its antithesis should be cause for alarm
Damage and devastation due to lockdown action
Dwarf viral rates and deaths by comparison

Magnified false positives using PCR approach
Keep up the pretence, no fear of reproach
Stay Indoors >Protect the NHS> Save Lives
These slogans are weapons akin to knives

Test, track and trace, mass vaccinations bring glory
Yet true numbers never printed, tell a different story
To question the propaganda, deceit and lousy data
Defines you as a conspiracy theorist or perpetrator

Who should we believe, there seems only one voice
Powerful media, which dictates and suppresses choice
Brave whistleblowers who dare speak their reality
Blocked, discredited, erased, along with humanity
We must stay confined, 'til the virus is low
But where did all the other diseases go?
Only room for one certified cause of death
Earns more money, who cares about final breath

Audacious, blatant infringement of human rights
New laws now overrule previous justice overnight
Families continually banned from visiting care homes
No hugs, goodbyes for loved ones, left to die alone

Coercion, deception, manipulation on a monumental scale
Anyone who questions can expect an arrest, maybe jail
Mandate police power, start knocking on front doors
Old norms now history, ever to return to our shores?

Dr Lisa Hutchinson February 2021

A Parallel Universe by Caroline Sargeant

I saw the footage being shared online,
peeking at grandma through the looking glass,
hands pressed to window.......no touching is fine?
Vectors of disease, unless you had a pass.

A parallel universe is what I saw,
humanity reduced to testing and tracing.
PCR test positive, even if you were well,
what deadly disease was this we were facing?

The TV screen said there was much to fear.
Lockdown, stay safe, don't question the narrative...
but covid and flu IFR were alike, it appears,
yet following rules, until Vax was imperative!

Loved ones dying alone during lockdowns,
bereft of the human touch to ease the passing.
How did we ever agree to that?
A parallel universe.....deeply disturbing!

I looked on in horror with freedoms curtailed.
Dissenting voices, smeared and cast aside.
Media said "follow the science" but science failed,
if you can't test the theories, truth is denied.

Children were shields to protect the adults.
Masked up, shut down, a tragedy unfolding,
ignore their pain....just follow the cult,
my mind was distressed, a sense of foreboding!

My world view will never be the same again.
A parallel universe is what I saw,
a few, controlled the many, which seemed insane,
reminiscent of Orwell's 1984.

Caroline Sargeant 2023.

The Killing Years by David Vance

I never saw it coming, I once had faith in science
But after a three-year nightmare, I now trust self-reliance;
Killer doctors pushing jabs, vile politicians demanding your compliance.
The only course left to us was to forge a new alliance.

At first, they came for the old and frail, those who were most defenceless
But the quest to injure, maim and kill was strong and equally relentless.
"Roll up your sleeve and take the shot, it's safe and 100% effective"
The lies they told, which the media sold, were shockingly seductive

I never took their toxic poison; I was proud to stand against it
I never outsourced my thinking to some clowns spouting bullshit
The time when come when they are judged and great will be there fear
And we'll remember what they did to us all in the cruel killing years.

David Vance

Cell For Sale by M Joseph Burt

Cell for sale
I'm selling the cell,
You're forewarned It's a four-walled
Living hell
The aspect is irrelevant,
And the vista as well,
Whichever way that you are facing
As you're pacing,
You can never tell,

The toilet is open plan,
And yet it is quite discreet
As the cell, is, well, private,
You have your own en suite,
And parking's a dream,
There's no need to compete,
As there's no street, it's wherever you park your feet,

The soft sell is that it comes
At a competitive price,
Stuck in your head
A prisoner of your own advice,
Never think once,

But always think twice,
And on second thoughts,
Let anxiety entice,

I'm selling the cell
Yeah I'm moving out
Out of my head,
And out and about,
I'm leaving behind
The lock and the key,
And the prison of anxiety
And the jailer who I now realise
Has been me.

M Joseph Burt 7th February 2023
For more poetry by this author please see his books:

Closing the Lid by the BARRED BARD

To all my fellow countrymen, my neighbours and my kin,
Pandora's box has blown its lid, its demons in full spin.
These demons aren't fictitious, they're living with us now,
They're dressed in suits from institutes, so 'holier-than-thou'.

They come with great credentials, so they're bound to be believed
And judging by their roadmap there is lots that they've achieved.
That's why so many countries are all doing just the same
Where their leaders spout catchphrases like a 'Simple Simon' game

The government is killing us and too few seem to care
They're jabbing children from year 1, how do they even dare!
But that's the thing with psychopaths, they think they can just do
So, if you don't wake to close this lid…
They'll soon be killing **you**!

THE BARRED BARD September 2023

David stood up by June Slater

David stood up
Ready to be counted
The research was scant
The fear mounted
The vaccine was out
The product was touted
Try to resist
And you'd soon be outed

Shame on you the crowd did roar
Big pharma sat back
Seeing profits soar
Take it now
You need it to travel
Heart attacks, strokes as the narrative unravels

The Doc stood firm
He took the abuse
The drug they sold us, not fit for use
Tested for weeks when it's normally years
The side effects mount
With the shedding of tears

I listened to the Doc who risked his career.
I didn't get vaxxed and I'm healthy, I'm here
I didn't listen to the scientists who stood to gain
I listened to the ones prepare for the pain

June Slater

Shropshire Boy by Andrew Horler

It's time to see clearly; are you waking up?
This veil of evil; time to take it off.
I still grieve the; life I used to have
But now I see clearly; I've a second chance

Westminster theatre; are you partied out?
Hospital theatres; full of Midazolam
Freedom does not start; at the needle's end
Safe and effective; what a fucking scam

Oooohhhhhh can you feel it now
Oooohhhhhh can you feel it now

Freedom is precious
Let's take a stand
Coz we are the ninety nine percent
I know it's scary
I understand
I'm always here to hold your hand

Sometimes I play chess; in the chequered sky
They say they are contrails; it's just another lie
They mask and they muzzle us; trying to keep us quiet
Well I've got four words for you; we will not comply

They man make disasters; then they smack our ass
They're getting as common; as DEW on autumn
grass
They traffic our children; all part of their plan
Don't wait 'til it's your child; before you take a stand.

Andrew Horler

A Poem by Tanya R

The thing that changed our world
When it really shouldn't have
Is the Covid pandemic and the vaccine
That made so many glad.

Little did they know that the war had begun
And all of those who spoke the truth,
They decided they should shun
Ivermectin as a respected course
Of treatment for Covid,
Not just for a horse.
Health Canada , and the FDA
Made it sound like you might start chewing hay.

The Media of course jumped on the tale
And 90% of the population decided to bale
The main stream medical used hospital protocol
The outcomes of which have now been seen by all
Remdesivir was just certain death
While paxlovid was sorta like no breath.

Within 7 to 10 days Covid would reoccur
But that's OK Your vaccinated,
So you felt really safe and sure

Morphine was given to finish the old
But it was from Covid every death we were told

Put on your mask to stop the spread
Even though each hole
Lets through ten Covid spore threads

We needed two weeks to stop the spread
Now it's four years And still
The vaccinated are dead
Both buy the shot, in two ways
The vaccine injury
And your natural immunity decay.

Our inflation went high, as did interest rates
As you laid down your morals and science
For a slice of the cake
You dehumanized people and thought it ok
But one day in the future you will have to pay.

Tanya R.

What a Mystery by N Turner

January two thousand and twenty,
Corona virus had arrived.
It spread like wildfire in plenty,
Told it was so deadly and lucky to survive.

Lockdown was harsh to reduce the spread,
Disabled & elderly told to shield.
No contact with anyone to reduce the dead,
As covid pneumonia was difficult to heal.

The vaccine came as saviour from grace,
Yet all administrations were masked to save their face.
It was experimental we took in trust,
To save the planet pandemic it was a must!

With hope & faith we trusted in doctors,
We took what was give just like sheep.
If we questioned it they just mocked us,
So secretly decided with a card to keep.

Only need two they said,
To go on holiday and be free,
I still can't believe how easily lead,
As we trusted those with a degree.

How we failed to see their wizardry,
Many more still got sick and died.
Doctors said " what a Mystery?"
They are now so ignorance & lied.

Have another booster as didn't last long,
Few started to question the science,
So doctors parroted disinformation as a new song,
Yet we know the harms & damage of their vaccines defiance.

It's safe and effective they said,
Yet won't say the adverse side effects?
We now know how dangerous from the increased dead,
All induced turbo cancer & heart attacks.

Now we stand together against mRNA,
Trust & faith has dwindled with this time,
With god narcissist egos that scientist like to play,
Some smart doctors stood up for our safety to expose the lie.

Doctors need to acknowledge this vital mistake,
As this was a deathly humanitarian crime.
The boosters are poisonous and demonic,
Data for 75yrs they wanted to hide.

More have awoke to this evil endgame,
It's biological warfare unknown attack.
Many refused anymore just to stay sane,
There are Angel doctors that have out back

They stood up to big pharma,
Government and close colleagues too.
They kept their oath of do no harm,
Criticised and lost their jobs all to keep on
protecting YOU!

So this IQ test is just for the smartest,
As only they against all odds will survive.
As government haven't fooled the best,
Who have noticed who's injured and died.

Not all hero's wear capes,
The rare doctors who care shine so bright.
We will keep saying No that evil GPs hate,
For all health safety and sanity we must fight.

N Turner

Boo Hoo by Dr Billy Ralph

WEF, WEF said Lev. Lev is happy. Look his tail is wagging.

Oink Oink said the doctor, lifting his head from the trough. The doctor is happy. Lev is his friend.

Baa, Baa said the people. The people think they are happy. The people like Lev. Lev will protect them.

Cock-a-doodle-do said the policeman. The policeman is happy. Lev feeds him lots of corn.

Meow, meow said the Pharmer. Lev likes the Pharmer. The Pharmer likes Lev. Together they will do great things.

Moo, Moo said the scientist. The scientist is happy. The Pharma is kind to the scientist.

Buzz, buzz said the journalist, softly. The journalist is happy. He doesn't want to disturb Lev and the Pharmer.

Boo, hoo said the children. The children are crying. Why?

WEF, WEF said Lev as he shrugs and the Pharmer grins.

Dr Billy Ralph

A Visit from December 2019 by Erika Loch

'Twas the last New Year's Eve, before shit got weird.
Covid was stirring, but hadn't fully appeared
Flights were booked freely, and without fanfare
We took it for granted, we could go anywhere !

Children would play, without any fear
That they would kill Granny if they were near
While visions of sugar plums danced in their heads
Before they were charged with stopping the spread.

We went about our business, with love and with care
The promise of a new year, dancing in the air
When out east in China, a storm had been brewing
We carried on, as if nothing was doing.

Away to our parties, our families and friends
Not knowing it'd be some time before we saw them again.
The moon on the crest of what was to come
A story foretold, but only to some.

When what to our wandering hearts did appear
We wouldn't know yet, it wasn't at all clear
We looked at our phones, and clinked our glasses
It was perfectly natural, to be in the masses.

We kissed and we hugged with reckless abandon
Not fearing the germs of beloved companions
Now, freedom! now, love! now, reflection and hope!
The new year is here, and it's going to be dope!

To the top of any mountain! To planting a new tree!
We planned ahead, as if we were free!
We buried old hatchets, and made resolutions
Excitement, desire, and future solutions.

So much ahead, an historical year!
The year of 20/20 – but not a thing was clear. We
didn't yet know, what was coming our way
We knew f*** all, suffice it to say.

We took in champagne, and decorated our faces
We sang and we danced without track or traces!
We went to the pub without QR codes
Without rapid testing, we opened our abodes.

We hugged and kissed strangers, not knowing their
status
A toast to good health! Before there was malice.
Before there was a needle that would come between
us
A time before now, when we met with freeness.

Our problems felt real, though many were petty
We have learned by now, if we didn't already
Time is precious, our years fill the album
Time is fleeting, and little is random.

'Twas the last New Year's Eve, before shit got weird
Covid was coming, and designed to be feared
But we kept on going, not heeding the warnings
With the same trust and hope that comes every
morning.

Because we are human, 'tis our natural state
To live life with ease, despite and through hate.
When we dig deep, we remember who we are
Brothers and sisters – sun, moon and stars.

So let us take heart, and gather our strength
And remember to strive for the highest wavelength
Woke isn't awake, and freedom isn't free
Gone are the days of being spiritually lazy.

Gone are the days of innocence, again
History repeats, and still, we don't learn
They signal their virtue with shields that don't work
They do not see, they are serfs de la cirque.

Draw down your guards and keep faith in your heart
Do not forget, Humanity is Art.
'Tis a new start again, and all through the land
The human spirit rises, at its own command.

Switch off the news, and turn down the fear
Let Love be the new variant, of this next year.
As we forge ahead and out of the blight
Happy new year to all, may this year bring you light.

By Erika Loch

Reflection by Dr Anon Doctor

In March 2020 I knew: "I see you....you pandemic of fear". But we don't live in fear we live by faith. "Perfect love casts out all fear". Switch off the tv. The BBC is clearly pushing terror propaganda.

Once you see it, you can't unsee it. Why does nobody see it? Why are friends trying to educate me on how on earth lockdown works against a tiny airborne virus?

It's the dumbest idea ever; it will destroy society, the economy, livelihoods, my children's lives and special experience milestones.

Once you see it you can't unsee it. Lies. Everywhere.

A fearful friend who I couldn't persuade, shared a psalm: Psalm 91. I laminated it and put one copy next to my bed and one in my office. It spoke comfort and faith to me through these dark years:

> Those who live in the shelter of the Most High will
> find rest in the shadow of the Almighty.
>
> This I declare about the Lord: He alone is my refuge,
> my place of safety; he is my God, and I trust him.
>
> For he will rescue you from every trap and protect
> you from deadly disease.

He will cover you with his feathers. He will shelter you with his wings.

His faithful promises are your armor and protection.

Do not be afraid of the terrors of the night, nor the arrow that flies in the day.

Do not dread the disease that stalks in darkness, nor the disaster that strikes at midday.

Though a thousand fall at your side, though ten thousand are dying around you, these evils will not touch you.

Just open your eyes, and see how the wicked are punished.

If you make the Lord your refuge, if you make the Most High your shelter, no evil will conquer you; no plague will come near your home.

For he will order his angels to protect you wherever you go.

They will hold you up with their hands so you won't even hurt your foot on a stone.

You will trample upon lions and cobras; you will crush fierce lions and serpents under your feet!

The Lord says, "I will rescue those who love me. I will protect those who trust in my name.

When they call on me, I will answer; I will be with them in trouble.

I will rescue and honor them. I will reward them with a long life and give them my salvation."

Unable to talk to most friends and family without being attacked, I found new friends, and love and support in unexpected places.

There was no way they were going to stop me going to work, doing my job saving lives; not from "Covid" but from cancer, and the general surgery emergencies I managed day in day out.

The roads were empty. Eerie.

The carpark was half empty.

The hospital corridors empty. Eerie.

ICCU expanded. Theatre staff redeployed. First cancer-case I'd ever had postponed for lack of bed.

But we carried on. We treated cancers. In 2020, 3 of my post-op patients suddenly died of unexpected heart attacks…de-conditioned by lockdown, stricken by stress and fear?

I continued to meet with my faithful Christian brother and sister every Thursday to pray for our church and our nation and fight the darkness.

Then the real madness. Natural (real) immunity quashed. The vaccine saviour promises, the mantra, the hypnotising dogma and the religious ferver of the worshippers who swallowed the ridiculous old lie "safe and effective"...how could it possibly be so with warpspeed marketing...

"Why are all our patients scans coming back with clots?" - the admin staff could see whilst medical colleagues were blind...and then an unexpected Dr hero stood up. Steve James. On Sky TV. He Stood up. And 100k stood up. "No way". "Go away" we said. If it costs me my job so be it. My children are not having this and I am not having any more than that one AZ regret. Never would I accept experimental RNA. Coerced by two men I had trusted with spiritual authority "to love thy neighbour", and for the sake of alleviating the fears my patients might have that I could "put them at risk". Both mentors had failed the test; the ethical and moral test. So now I see you too. As for me and my house...

Anon Doctor

Uneasyjet by Steven Jackson

This holiday was the only time I gave in (to my family and the immovable Easyjet captain) to put a cloth mask on my chin. On the way out, a pair of underpants (clean) worn as a neck warmer and a large bag of peanuts kept the Karens at bay.

25 August 2020

I sit on an Easyjet night-flight back from Portugal.

As the light from the airport disappears I feel a growing uneasiness.

I sit with my mask dropping from my face Knowing the guards at the front of the plane are sat down and cannot see my misbehaviour.

I have the most uneasy feeling. It is, I imagine, something similar to that felt on the trains through Poland and Germany. We are a long way from that, but how sudden it is that we are here already.

The videos of police brutality in New Zealand, Australia and France passing without comment or condemnation from anyone in power or with influence. Silence from journalists. Silence from charities and churches, synagogues and mosques. Scientists muttering some minor dissent little more than a quibble, too worried for their career to worry about evidence anymore.

I am fearful for my children, who are 16 and 18. I am fearful for the sadness that is about to grip what we called Great Britain. For the splitting up of families, the depression and illness to be inflicted. For the struggle that life is becoming, but must become for as many of us as possible if our children are to know freedom and joy.

I sit with tears in my eyes. I will wipe them before this flight ends.

I am listening to what has been described as perhaps the most beautiful music ever written. I will take it as my inspiration but remind myself to switch to something more defiant and triumphant in mood. It is only in this moment that I realise that, for me at least, music is going to be important in this war as it has been to others in the past. I will fight tomorrow, the day after and for the next weeks and months and, if necessary, years. Our lives are not theirs to take away.

Steven Jackson

About Dr David Cartland

My name is Dr David Cartland and I am a GP based in Cornwall. My medical training was slightly unconventional in that I did a prior degree in Biomedical sciences and some medical research prior to starting the graduate medical programme so effectively 8 years of undergraduate training. Graduation was a proud moment for me and my family as I come from a working-class background and was the first Doctor across generations of my family. One of the memories of the graduation ceremony is when we all joined together in reciting the Hippocratic Oath where one thing stood out to me from the oath to this day....Primum non nocere....first do no harm. Sadly this is being phased out of many UK graduation ceremonies.

I decided to become a doctor and more importantly a GP because I relish the challenges of primary care and being a generalist. More importantly I love to practice holistic medicine and wanted to follow the path of the old-fashioned cradle to grave 'Family doctor' sadly now of yesteryear where you follow a patient from birth to being elderly and understand people's illness in context of their psychosocial background.

In 2020 when the pandemic was announced I remember signing a waiver of liability at my surgery to join the fight against this unknown disease despite being medically exempt from attending face to face due to my asthma. My initial approach to the pandemic was observational and seeing the disparity from what I encountered in hospitals and my practice/urgent care work compared to the MSM coverage which was starkly polar opposite. It was genuinely the quietest 6-12 months of my career. I moved from the Midlands to Cornwall for a better work life balance just as vaccination against covid-19 was being discussed. I have been fully vaccinated for all other communicable disease in the past and regrettably took two covid jabs (the latter under high amounts of coercion). Training had taught me never to question vaccine safety as this was career suicide, they were safe and effective across the board no questions asked!

When the first and second jab programme started I didn't see that much in regard of vaccine harms but when the booster campaign started I saw exponential increases in patient harm from a breadth of new onset co-morbidity. At the same time I was witnessing many strange public health policies being invoked as well as a trend that most people who were vaccinated were incessantly catching covid time and time again. None of this made sense and I started my more detailed research around Autumn 2021 and started to attempt to raise alarm bells in my practice and locality. Sadly despite presenting data and published studies the immediate reaction towards me was that I was a (vaccinated) anti-vaxxer (despite it not even being a conventional vaccine), conspiracy theorist and had somehow lost the plot. I was advised that despite my concerns I should 'keep my head down and shrug my shoulders' by a senior colleague.

This appalled me. We are duty bound as doctors to follow GMC guidance on things such as informed consent, Good medical practice, Duty of candour and confidentiality. All I could see was that my colleagues across the NHS seemed to have forgotten this strict guidance seemingly overnight. I decided to speak out and the rest is history.

I tried to contact MSM channels and newspapers but never got a response, so I decided to contact a multitude of non mainstream media outlets and did interviews to escalate my concerns. As my position as one of very few doctors speaking out grew, so too did the trolling and online censorship increase. Not long after my initial essay 'Breaking the Silence' went viral, in quick succession I was swiftly banned from every single social media platform. This was such sinister development. What happened to debate and discussion which even up to this very day I have lacked engagement with? This was also happening to many of my colleagues that had dared to raise alarm bells.

At this point, I seemed to be gaining a negative reputation locally for asking questions, presenting data and evidence from journals contrary to the popular narrative of safe and effective. To say otherwise was considered blasphemy and as myself and other colleagues have since realised a huge risk to our medical careers secondary to GMC investigation and coordinated online abuse/trolling and medical establishment cancel culture.

It has been a very challenging, surreal time of my career, seemingly in trouble and risking my medical license for having genuinely held un-rebutted ethical and safety concerns, for promoting evidence-based medicine and helping those injured by the vaccine amongst other crimes. Yet I have faith in the Lord and belief that the truth must and **will** come out.

God bless you.

David.

Printed in Great Britain
by Amazon

33849026R00086